AUTOMATIC NATURAL WEIGHT LOSS SYSTEM

"Healthier Living Series"

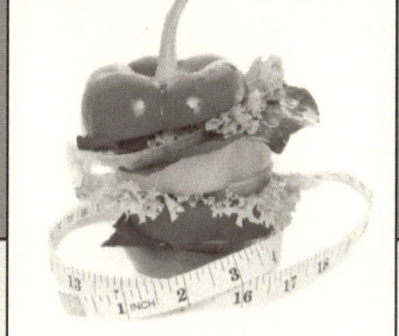

Franklin Gillette

Automatic Natural Weight Loss System

Automatic Natural Weight Loss System

By: Franklin Gillette

Distributed by: Lulu Press

Copyright

Automatic Natural Weight Loss System

Second Edition

Notice

This book is intended as a reference volume and neither as a
medical text nor to give medical advice. This book is not
intended to prescribe medical treatment, heal, or cure
diseases. It is for informational and educational purposes
only. The information within is designed to help you make
better decisions regarding your health and diet choices. The
result will speak for itself. Always consult your doctor or
seek the advice of a professional medical practitioner before
beginning any type of weight loss or diet plan.

More from This Author

- **Compatibility: Code of Harmony for Love and Unity "Happier Relationship Series"**
- **The Street Knowledge Family Guide of Drug Prevention "Healthier Living Series"**
- **How to Protect Yourself, Family, Property and Valuables from Crime in Public or at Home "Household Solutions Series"**
- **The Secrets of Concentration and Mental Rejuvenation "Self Improvement Series"**
- **How to Make Extra Money at Home Right now "Greater Wealth Series"**
- **How to Live Life Happily After Divorce "Happier Relationship Series"**

Table of Contents

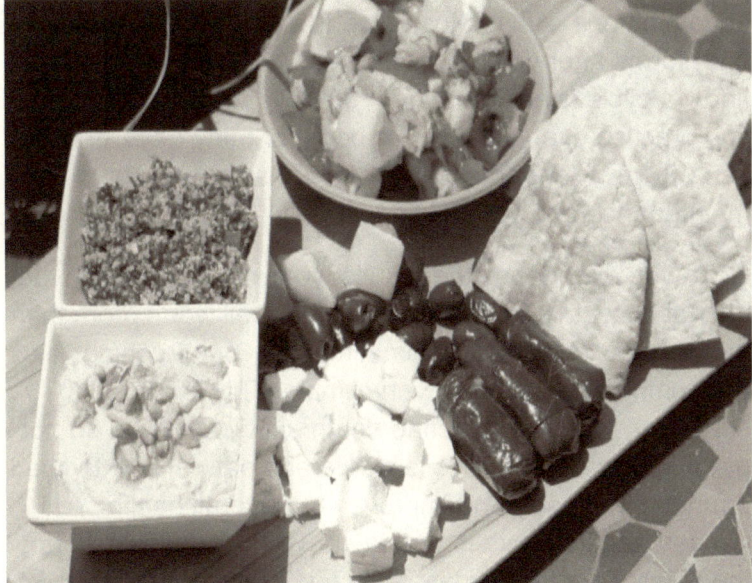

Foreword

I have devoted my life to healthy living and sharing these principles with others in hopes we all can have a healthy and more productive lifestyle. I was inspired to write this book and other books by the many people who encouraged me to put the knowledge I have accumulated through the years on paper. I answered the call and the need to produce an extremely factual and helpful book concerning weight loss and the proper steps to achieve your renewed health.

This Book guarantees to break some bad habits by learning your body's natural cycles and rhythms and becoming one with it. Most experts say a habit (good or bad) forms after doing it for at least 21 days straight. We know a cycle is half an hour or 30 days for completion. If you practice everything in this book for thirty days straight, you will have formed a good habit of natural weight maintenance and you will keep it off!

Once you experience the results, you will wonder why you did not know this before. This book is well worth more than the cost as you will see. Sometimes we look for things that are complicated, and it is very simple. This is not a diet scam or a "starve yourself to death" diet where you do not get proper nutrients. This is a safe and natural way to shed pounds effortlessly and improve your overall health. You will see results way before thirty days if you follow this to the letter. Truthfully, in less than two weeks you should experience more energy, better sleep, and a more positive outlook.

Introduction

Have you tried diet plan after diet plan and gotten the same results? Have you lost weight and then gained it right back? Are you tired of eating less because you thought it would help you lose weight? Well throw those diets and myths out the window! Most diets are the reason you cannot keep the weight off and actually keep you fat. Another problem is losing the weight then gaining it right back. According to the latest health statistics, over two thirds of Americans are overweight or obese.

We have a solution. *Automatic Natural Weight Loss System* is an automatic fat burning system that you can apply immediately. That is right, when you are finished reading this book, you will be able to apply the time-tested secrets to weight loss and maintenance. Whether you want to lose 5 pounds or 50 pounds, *Automatic Natural Weight Loss System* will help you achieve your weight loss goals. In fact, you do not even have to apply the whole book to lose weight. You can apply a chapter at a time and get excellent results. Your body works in cycles. When you dishonor those cycles, your body responds in weight gain and disease.

Not only will I provide guaranteed fat burning secrets, I will also provide worldwide proven secrets that other cultures practice to maintain their natural weight. Have you ever seen an overweight person on the walls of Egypt or in hieroglyphics? I do not remember seeing many or any at all. Obviously, a system was in place to solve and avoid obesity. We have generally removed ourselves from our natural cycles and nature. This book is the most logical and practical way to address not only losing weight, but also burning fat. When you are finished with this book, you will improve your overall health because holistic health is the foundation you will put in action. You will not find the combination of principles anywhere else except in this book.

This book is all you need as a pinpointed no nonsense guide to automatic fat burning. You will not have to spend extra money on expensive memberships, products, surgeries, shots, or other nonsense. This book contains the newest principles on losing weight and burning fat by addressing it holistically and completely. You will wonder why you have not heard of this sooner. It will make so much sense because it gets right to the point. You do not need a 200 page complicated manual. You need a simple and practical way to finally burn that fat! Have fun with this book, as you will learn how to live better and look good at the same time.

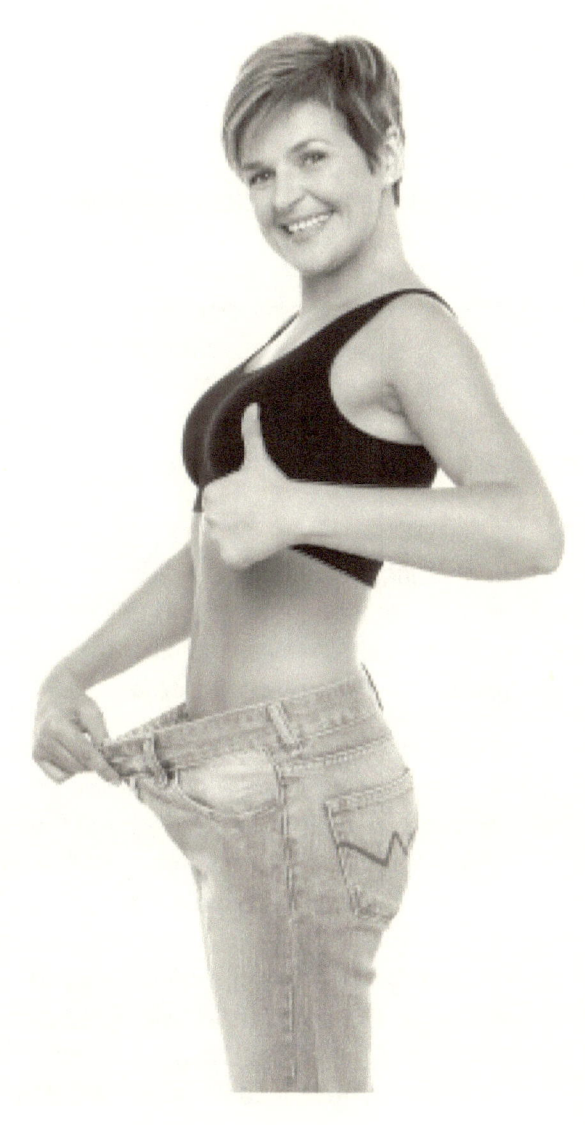

Chapter 1

What is Holistic Health?

Holistic health is a concept in medical practice upholding that all aspects of people's needs, psychological, physical and social, and mentally should be taken into account and seen as a whole. As defined above, the holistic view on treatment is widely accepted in medicine.

Holistic Health

[1] A different definition, claiming that disease is a result of physical, emotional, spiritual, social and environmental imbalance, is used in alternative medicine. [2]
From Wikipedia, The free encyclopedia

The Ancient Egyptians first practiced holistic health, sometimes-spelled wholistic health, thousands of years ago. When referencing the Ancient Egyptians, one must be careful not to categorize them as one people. For example, the Egyptians referenced in the bible were different from Pre-Dynastic Egyptians. That is very important because people do not identify with Ancient Egypt because they think they were all one people. There was Predynastic Egypt, Dynastic Egypt, and Post Dynastic Egypt with many invasions in between. These invasions caused differences in people, customs, and even practices. The people and the environment changed. You would not put all Americans into one pot and judge them.

For example, you would not judge the actions of a fraternity today (doing harmful acts) with the actions of the fraternity in its founding years. You would be considering different people, different factors, influences, morals, and much more. This is necessary to express because The Ancient Egyptians, known for their holistic healing methods and health practices, aligned with natural methods. We do not want to discard them because of misinformation. They did not just consider an ailing body part. Instead, they considered the physical, spiritual, emotional, and mental body as one to be treated as a whole. This brought balance to the body and not just a part of the body. This is holistic health.

If you had three children you would not take care of just one, you would take care of all three. The same is with the body, as you would bring the whole body into balance. That is why it's called the ears, eyes, nose, and throat doctor. If you are dreaming, your physical body is laying in bed. What part of you is participating in the dream? Now you see there is more to you that exists than just the physical. Holistic Health deals with the whole you, not just a part of you. Its remedies help the body from ailments and dis-ease through foods, herbs, sound, touch, scents, energy, sight, and more.

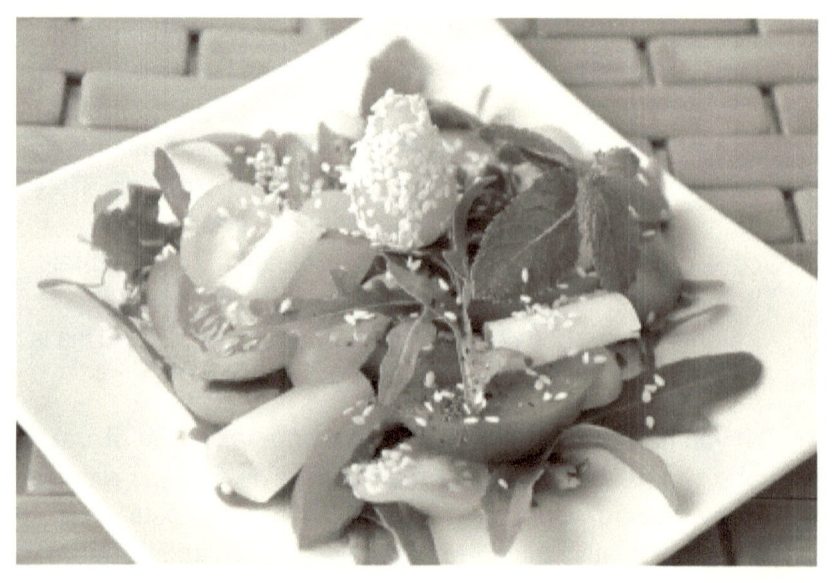

Chapter 2

Diets are Shortcuts to Holistic Health

What is the Difference Between Holistic Health and Medicine Practiced Today?

The difference between holistic health and medicine practiced today is like night and day. Holistic Health deals with the cause, and medicine today usually deals with the symptoms. Why take medicine to stop the pain, nausea, headaches, etc. from the flu when you can deal with the cause of the flu directly without any more side effects. Holistic Health restores the body part, system, or organ back to its normal function naturally by bringing balance. Medicine usually stops the effects of the ailment that masks the real issue. This is why people stay on blood pressure medicine or insulin for years with the condition not getting any better. Holistic Health is natural and works with the body's cycles. Everything in nature works in cycles.

What are the Results for Not Practicing Holistic Health?

The result for not practicing holistic health is detrimental over time. The ailments or disease of the body is untreated because of treatments with medicine and over the counter drugs. You may not notice the damage immediately, but it will happen over time like a slow poison. Most people are not born with cavities, high blood pressure, breast cancer, prostate cancer, gout, and other ailments. It happens over time because of not keeping the whole body or holistic body healthy. When people do not practice holistic health, the condition or ailment you suffer from usually goes unnoticed and gets worse over time.

Is Holistic Health the Same as Dieting?

The definition of diet is as follows:

Diet (dīʹĭt)
n. The usual food and drink of a person or animal.
A regulated selection of foods, as for medical reasons or cosmetic weight loss.
Something used, enjoyed, or provided regularly: subsisted on a diet of detective novels during his vacation.

adj. Of or relating to a food regimen designed to promote weight loss in a person or an animal: the diet industry.
Having fewer calories.
Sweetened with a no caloric sugar substitute.
Designed to reduce or suppress the appetite: diet pills; diet drugs.

v., -et·ed, -et·ing, -ets.

v.intr To eat and drink according to a regulated system. This is especially done to lose weight or control a medical condition.

v.tr. To regulate or prescribe food and drink for.
[Middle English diete, from Old French, from Latin diaeta, way of living, diet, from Greek diaita, back-formation from diaitāsthai, to live one's life, middle voice of *diaitān*, to treat.]
American Heritage Dictionary

As you can see, dieting means many different things according to the many definitions but it is not the same as holistic health. Dieting usually only addresses the physical body and not the spiritual, mental, or emotional body.

Holistic health is in a sense more related to the etymology (origin) of diet. The etymology of diet was a way of living or a way of life. It then spiraled into the thousands of diets today that range from the lemonade diet to the liquid diet. Holistic Health deals with the physical, mental, spiritual, and emotional body. Diets usually deal only with the physical body.

What is Wrong With Diets and Why Don't They Work?

Diets are usually incomplete. There are thousands of diets all claiming to be the best. If they do not fit into the body's natural cycles then it is incomplete. It usually deals with one aspect of losing weight that is abstaining from certain foods, eating only certain foods or liquids, or calorie watching. In addition, when you do this your physical body is usually deficient in nutrients and this affects your body. If you are deficient in nutrients, your body's organs and systems cannot work properly. This results in your body demanding more of what is necessary to replace what was lost and have some for reserve. The reserve is what you do not need. We call it fat!

Another problem with dieting is that it is usually unnatural how fast the weight is lost or the methods used. Most diets may cause you to lose weight for a moment in time but you usually are deficient in another area because of ignoring total health. That is why you see someone who has lost weight and discover that other health issues are present. If you keep letting your gas in your car run low then eventually all the deposits in your gas tank will start to go through your engine and cause harm over time. This is the same with your body. If you lose the weight and do not eliminate the toxins and address the other health issues, you will end up with more health problems to overcome later on.

Dieting is not the key because it is not holistic. It does not address the emotional, spiritual, and mental bodies. If not addressed, then you will gain it right back with the "seesaw" effect. Your weight goes down and then it goes right back up. People do not understand why that happens but it is very simple holistically why that happens. Your body seeks balance so if you starve or limit yourself unnaturally, your body will have urges and impulses to put back what was missing before. You can go on a lemonade diet, but what happens when you get off the diet? You gain it right back and your body is usually deficient in nutrition, which leaves you with other issues. Today, even most experts in the field are saying diets and fads do not work.

Chapter 3

Holistic Health and Diet Myths

Is Holistic Health and *Automatic Natural Weight Loss System* the same?

No, it is not. The *Automatic Natural Weight Loss System* utilizes holistic health to achieve its goal of fat burning and weight loss. Holistic health deals with more than just weight loss and weight control. Holistic health deals with disease prevention and restoration of the whole body and its natural functions.

Is it Necessary to Fast or Be a Vegetarian to Lose Weight?

No, it is not. Fasting for long periods is not healthy. Most people fast for health or religious reasons. It is healthy to fast at a certain time each week or month to give your digestive system a rest. Most times when you fast it eliminates toxins from the body and sometimes water weight is lost. Losing water weight and fat is very different. We are interested in losing the weight from fat, not just water. There are many types of vegetarians and studies show that it is healthier for you, but it is not necessary to lose weight. Many people lose weight every day that do not fast or practice vegetarianism.

Do the Boxed Celebrity Diets Work?

Those diets are expensive and you still have to buy the vegetables. You spend lots of money instead of saving your money and making better choices.

Why Don't I Just Get a B12 (Cobalamin or Cyanocobalamin) Shot?

Why spend all that money to do something that you can do naturally? It is the same reason why you do not take steroids! It is unnatural regardless of what they say. I am not concerned with what so-called health professionals have to say claiming its harmless and safe. They have not cured any major diseases today, so what can they say is good or bad for you? Medicine only masks the real issue.

Holistic Health is the only remedy that safely and naturally helps maintain and restore good health. Holistic health addresses the total body, instead of listening to people saying medicine is safe. They also said Viagra was safe when it came out. It is always great in the beginning until the side effects and problems show up later. Did they also say that when they were prescribing Viagra and the other medications that are either bad or getting recalled? Those things are irreversible. We always want quick results and that is why people and bad habits have eliminated the natural cycles of the body, diet, digestion, and ultimately the natural laws of life.

People have stepped in and created shortcuts to capitalize off people's emotions, thoughts, and insecurities. The fast food industry is a result of saving time and being convenient, yet it is unhealthy for you. Microwaves are the result of the same reasoning, and it too is unhealthy. Canned and boxed dinners are in that category, designed to make large companies extremely profitable from people's shortcomings. They are not concerned with your well-being. The real problems occur when you interfere with the natural cycles of life and your body. Your body responds with ailments and disease. It may not respond right away either.

People want the B12 shot because it is a shortcut like steroids. It will affect your body negatively later. To give your body part of what it needs instead of the whole food, plant, root, or herb, is part of the solution. You need whole solutions for a whole body. There are supporting systems and elements in foods and herbs the same way you have supporting organs, tissues, and systems in your body. This is the same throughout nature and the universe. It is funny how you can overdose on Vitamin B supplements, but not from food. The list of side effects than can occur from the B12 shot are: Diarrhea, anxiety and panic attacks, heart palpitations, insomnia, breathing problems, chest pain, headache, joint pain, hives, rash, and swollen skin. Of course, these symptoms go unchecked the same way other warning signals from our body go unchecked.

Most do not know these Vitamin B12 shots contain preservatives that do damage to your body over time that leads to problems later. Is it really worth the risk? You can solve the problems of obesity and being overweight by simply changing your food choices and practicing the principles in this book. It is not something new, but we are just reminding you. So if you must take B-12, take the vitamin or eat the foods rich in Vitamin B-12. Vegetarians or Vegans can eat fortified cereals, drinks, spreads, and other fortified products if there is a deficiency.

What are the Dangers of Getting a Tummy tuck?

I will not spend too much time addressing this because it should be somewhat obvious. For starters, it costs normally $2,000-$10,000 to get this type of surgery done. Did I say surgery? Yes I did. Having someone cut into your body instead of just following simple health principles to lose weight naturally is dangerous. The emotional and mental body is out of balance causing the physical result. Holistic healing solves those issues first and then the physical is sure to follow. Getting a tummy tuck interferes with the body's natural cycles. In the future years, the body does not hold it up. Save your money and do it the right way. Many movie stars and actors do it the right way to get into a certain physical shape for a role and so can you!

I Work a Night Shift Job and Can't Seem to Lose Weight?

This is a common problem for many because the natural body's biorhythms are "thrown off" because you are awake when you should be resting. Because of this, cravings are increased which will interfere with your elimination system. Your body is eliminating whatever it did not use from the assimilation (nutrients used in the body from eating) process. You can still burn fat and lose the weight using The *Automatic Natural Weight Loss System*. All you have to do is plan and organize more than the average person organizes until your system is in place.

For example, you cannot eat your dinner at 1:00 a.m. because it would be interfering with your body's elimination cycle. This will actually feed and increase fat cells. If you must eat during these night hours then it should be fruits or vegetables that are water producing and juicy when bitten into. This is safe to eat after hours because it does not take much to digest and is less harmful on the system.

Examples of safe foods are melons, tomatoes, salads, pineapples, cucumbers, grapes, and other water-type foods. If you bring this to your job, it will eliminate the urge to eat vending machine food, fast food, or food too heavy on the system such as dinner food. If you need to bring pre-packaged fruit or vegetables to your job, that will help. Even bringing a nutrient rich smoothie or shake is beneficial too. Drinking plenty of water is helpful because it will help your body during the elimination cycle. Your larger or main meals will take place when you arise from your nightshift rest. Your body is waiting for nutrients and replenishing at that time.

Getting your exercise in during the night shift job should be easy too as well as energizing. During your break or during the shift at work, find time to walk, stretch, and exercise. If you can do 30 minutes then you will really benefit and burn those fat cells, but if you can only do 10 minutes then it can also help. You do not have to join a gym if you are lacking in time. Be creative and turn wherever you are into a gym. This is important to stimulate the cells that will replace the fat cells. So yes, you can lose weight if you work a night shift job or even two jobs. The key to your success is to prepare and organize more proficiently than the average person. Great decisions and preparation will help you burn those fat cells just as everybody else can.

How is Weight Gained and How is Weight Lost?

Weight is gained in muscle mass, fat deposits, and water weight. People who gain fat-related weight can do so by eating more food, becoming less active, or both. When energy intake exceeds energy expenditure, the body can store the excess energy in a dense high-energy form as fat. One pound of fat represents 3,500 calories, so over time excessive energy intake and lack of exercise contributes to fat gain and obesity. If you eat more than you exercise then you have a great chance of turning that food into fat.

When the body does not know what to do with the excess food, it becomes waste and is stored as fat cells. So actually, an overweight person is full of waste and cannot assimilate vitamins and minerals properly. This means the overweight person is suffering from malnutrition! It sounds odd but if you consider the facts, it is true. If your body is not getting proper nutrition, it stores food instead of utilizing food for its nutrients. Therefore, your body is always in a hungry state. The organs, glands, and systems cannot do its job because of the malnutrition and abuse.

Weight loss occurs when a person is in a state of negative energy balance. This is when the body is exerting more energy (working, moving, action, high metabolism) than it is consuming (food or supplements). It will use stored reserves from fat or muscle that gradually leads to weight loss. There are other ways in which weight is gained and lost ranging from medicine intake reactions to under/overactive glands in the body which is the reason why you can't lose weight. This is why it is very necessary to find out your personal assessment from a holistic health consultation. This is discussed later in this book.

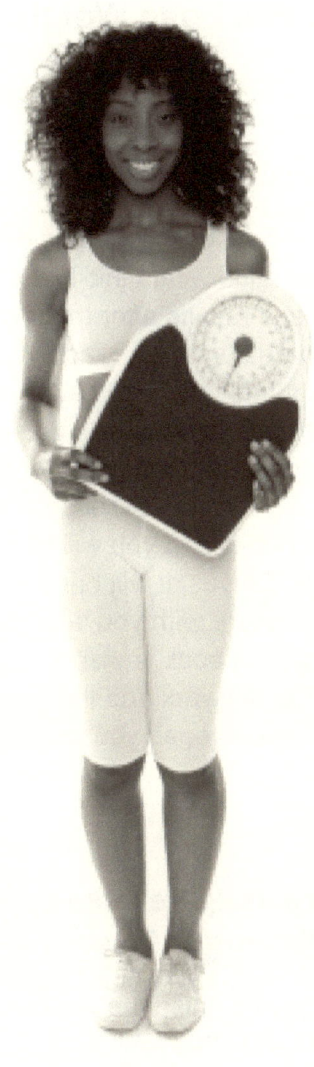

Chapter 4

Why you Will Lose Weight With This System

Is This Book Guaranteed to Bring Me Results?

If you truly follow the guidelines in this book by first studying the information within this book then putting it to practice, you will see results after the first week and then each week afterwards until you reach your natural body weight. Many diets and fads only cause you to lose water weight. This water weight is usually gained back over time. Because we approach fat burning holistically, the weight will stay off. This will happen because you will have built up a system of good habits and you will know how to stay holistically healthy. So yes, it will bring you results with all the secrets we will share with you later on in this book. This small yet practical book is well worth more than its weight in gold! This will work and the good thing is your overall health will improve, as you leave no stone unturned.

Will This System Help Reverse Some of My Other Ailments or Disease?

Yes, it will! People who finish the *Automatic Natural Weight Loss System* find that if they suffer from other conditions, it improves drastically or is sometimes even reversed or eliminated. Some of those conditions are High Blood Pressure, Arthritis, Diabetes, Gout, Crohn's Disease, Allergies, and more.

Can I Use Your System if I'm Pregnant?

It is perfect for pregnancy with the exception of Step 2 that is the colon cleanse and detox. You do not want to colon cleanse or detox during pregnancy. You can eat the right foods that are cleansing to achieve the same results. Most can use this system to lose the weight after pregnancy as well. Your hormones will not function in balance so Dandelion and Red Raspberry teas are excellent during your pregnancy to help with the balance.

Is This the Best Weight Loss System on the Market Today?

This is by far the best weight loss system on the market today because it is the most unique. This is a system that is not new, but rather renewed. This system represents the principle of "know thyself". There is not a system that approaches weight loss in the manner that we present to you. We feel simple facts with a practical system will help you faster. It utilizes the principles of the Ancient Egyptians and the cycles of the body, which were the first holistic health practitioners. Our system guarantees weight loss through fat reduction and you will not gain it back because of the holistic health support system in place. There is no system in place today that we know of that has so many simple facts that deal with the cycles of the body, holistic health, and ancient practices. We know of no system or diet program in place that will help you lose weight in the most natural and practical very possible.

Can Anyone Use Your System?

Yes! There are no restrictions because you are not doing anything other than putting your body back in balance with its natural systems and rhythms. This will actually improve your overall health with how simple it is.

Why Don't More People Know About This System?

People are unaware of our type of system because it would disrupt the economics of our society today. Look at the options we have today to destroy our health in the form of certain restaurants, fast food restaurants, medicines, and advertisements. You would see why our country has an average of an over 34% obesity rate. Why would "health and weight loss" be promoted if it will hit those same businesses in the pocket? That is why more people do not know about it. Holistic health keeps you away from the hospital or physician, reverses most ailments and disease, reduces or eliminates medicine intake, promotes healthy eating choices, and balances the total body affecting a shift and turn in our economy. The *Automatic Natural Weight Loss System* is written for your benefit, not the benefit of people's pockets. That is why more people do not know about these principles.

Can you Please Explain Your System?

It is a 9-step fat burning system geared towards addressing the body's cycles and bringing you back into balance with those systems. We chose the most practical and powerful fat burning tips known and put it into a system of nine. Why did we choose nine? We chose nine because there is no single digit bigger than nine. Six is a number symbolic of equality and imperfection. Seven is symbolic of perfection and nine is symbolic of completion. We do not want your weight loss to just be perfect; we want it to be complete!

Each step opens a door to the energy necessary to fight fat and restore your natural weight. We first remove all wastes and toxins from the body to lay a strong foundation. We then start helping you to lose weight physically, emotionally, spiritually, and mentally. We then put a holistic system in place with a system of renewal to keep it ongoing. There is a lot of misinformation out there concerning "weight loss and fat burning" so we eliminate all the fluff in our system and deal with only the facts. On top of all that, we put a series of health facts with powerful supporting facts to help provide you with tips you can put into practice immediately.

What if I don't finish all 9 steps?

If you do not finish all 9 steps, you will still see results. I have made what seems to be complex become very simple for you. You can put into practice as many steps as possible until you put all nine into practice. The steps are so easy that it will be impossible to not finish all 9 steps in 30 days. Then it will be completion! If you have problems with starting the system, then gain some momentum with some of the preceding tips and chapters.

The Quick Start Holistic Weight Loss program in this book is an excellent way to start, and see some immediate results. This will build your confidence to continue forward. The other chapters show international weight loss secrets, food combining, weight loss factors, and working with your body cycles to bring even greater overall results. These are all actions you can apply immediately for results and a boost of confidence. I included these helpful additions because I know some of you may want to start right away with something that is easy to do.

Most people want to lose weight, but just do not know where to begin. Moreover, they do not know why it is so hard. Others have lost hope and have accepted being overweight. I have presented the keys to reversing being overweight if you just take the time to put it in action. I have provided whole chapters of helpful hints to get you started with no hassle for those who say they do not have the time. Eventually you will have to complete the *Automatic Natural Weight Loss System* to get the full results. This is necessary because you will need a holistic path to completely losing weight with your whole body and not just your physical body. You will also need to restore your organs, systems, and glands because it is the reason why the body cannot assimilate the vitamins and minerals properly. I also followed with my very own *Automatic Natural Weight Loss System* for those who want more information, answers, and a system to follow. There is no excuse anymore.

You may have to stop eating what you are used to eating, but you can replace it with real food! Eating real food is less expensive than processed or hybrid food. Most hybrid foods (processed foods) are full of sugar and/or salt anyway. These two things cause the most problems in trying to lose weight anyway. You now have the tools necessary to start automatically lose some weight! Apply something every day so it becomes habit. Read your ingredient labels and choose the healthy alternative if necessary. Prepare and bring your food if you do not have healthy choices while you are away from home. It is hard but choose the grocery/supermarket over the restaurant and you will feel better. You will also see the weight disappear along with the "love handles" too! Just start with this book and apply it every day. You will see good habits formed and the body as proof of your healthier choices. Let us get started!

Chapter 5

Quick Start Holistic Weight Loss Automatic Fat Burning Solution

The purpose of this section is for those who want to add detail to their 9-step program. This will safely increase their automatic fat burning goals. You can also use this section alone to achieve great results as you incorporate your *Automatic Natural Weight Loss System*. If you are serious about weight loss and want to do it naturally, this is the immediate answer. You may not like what you have to do to accomplish immediate results, but then this is the reason why we are here in the first place.

I suggest you start from scratch and do an inventory of your food pantry/cabinets, refrigerator, and your freezer. Keep only the foods that are agreeable with the foods and suggestions in this book. The rest, get rid of it! Your health is more important than food that contributes to your weight gain! If you do not want to waste money, give it to charity or to a reputable cause so someone can use it. That blessing will come back to you. If you follow this section to the letter, you will be surprised of the immediate results. The results will grow like interest because you will reintroduce healthy eating back into your life with real foods!

This section will be addressing the physical body concerning holistic weight loss. Apply this to provide detail to your food choices in your diet plan. Incorporating these simple principles with step 4 of the *Automatic Natural*

Weight Loss System will fine-tune your goals naturally. Utilizing this section will bring you results alone but it does not alleviate the 9 step automatic fat burning process. You still need to colon cleanse, detox, get a holistic health consultation, and more. This is necessary to make this specific for you. It will help you know which foods are best for you to automatically burn fat and why. In addition, it will help you to eat the foods necessary to keep your pH balanced so your body will assimilate more nutrients from the foods you eat. Let us begin!

Quick Start Weight Loss in 5 Easy Steps

Step 1

First, Eliminate sugar foods from your diet. You can get it naturally in fruits. I am not just talking about eliminating donuts, cookies, cakes, pies and ice cream either. I'm talking about eliminating your so-called health foods such as: orange juice, whole wheat, ketchup, low fat salad dressing, low fat muffins, healthy cereal, and the list goes on. These foods have sugar listed on the ingredient labels. Sugar is also hidden as high fructose corn syrup! Eliminate high fructose corn syrup from your diet and you will automatically start to burn fat! They even put sugar into some canned vegetables! Read your labels, and you will see "sugar" and "high fructose corn syrup" on it. Put it back and choose the alternative that does not contain sugar or high fructose corn syrup on the ingredient label.

You are about to be shocked at the large amount of products that carry extra sugar and include high fructose corn syrup. You will see obesity was planned. You can eat sugar naturally in foods such as fruit, but when it too is overdone then there is a problem. It is a problem because it throws off your blood sugar level and sends it on a rollercoaster. It takes it high then it crashes. When it is high, your body releases a hormone called insulin that signals the body to <u>STORE</u> fat. Insulin is normal and good for the body because it regulates the blood sugar level and brings your blood sugar level down. When you release too much insulin, it takes your blood sugar level high, and then brings it down real low. This causes hunger, fatigue, and cravings, which causes you to eat more.

You definitely need insulin, but the roller coaster back and forth makes it impossible for fat burning because you are constantly storing fat and eating more until your pancreas goes berserk and stops producing insulin. It is called Diabetes. If you just avoid the foods that I mentioned above, your blood sugar level will not go out of whack, and you will start to automatically release the fat cells. The herb called Gymnema Sylvestre is excellent for stopping sugar cravings and blocks that sweet taste. Known as "the sugar killer", Gymnema Sylvestre can give you an even greater edge.

Step 2

Carbohydrates are not bad; it is just that none of them is the same. There are certain ones you need, and others you do not need. Some carbohydrates are not natural and cause the roller coaster with your blood sugar level. Whole wheat breads, grains, cereals, pastas, and crackers increase the insulin production and do not help burn fat just like the others. The Original and natural carbohydrates which became the alternatives today because of scarcity or price are: Sprouted grain, rice, amaranth, spelt, millet, quinoa, kamut, yam, and sweet potato are all examples of what you can make. Pasta, cereal, bread, crackers, and other nutritious meals can be made from the natural carbohydrates listed above. Sweet potatoes and yams are also real carbohydrates too. They are alkaline, and will help you automatically burn fat with the increased metabolic process taking place within your body. Good carbohydrates are also in (not hybrid) fruits and vegetables. Hybrid foods are acidic and should be limited in the diet. Big business and industry has stepped in and genetically altered some of our food and now you have seedless foods and other fruit and vegetables that were genetically altered.

Step 3

Do not be afraid to eat fat because it is not what makes you fat. When you eat fat, it increases the metabolic process used to automatically burn fat. The key is to know which fats to eat. Some cause you to store fat and others cause you to burn fat. Stay away from hydrogenated oils, canola oil, margarine, trans fats, and substituted butters. Because these fats are not real food, your body cannot use it and stores it as fat cells. Safe fats are fats that are naturally unprocessed, which burns fat off the body. This is opposite to the fats we have to choose from that are full of chemicals. Some are known as healthy and others are not in the health world, but these fats automatic cause fat burning: **real butter, whole eggs, coconut oil, olive oil, flax seed oil, avocados, and raw nuts to name a few.**

Step 4

Eat whole foods and stay away from the processed foods. Food in its natural form can be processed by every cell in the body. Processed food goes straight to the liver for processing. Processed foods usually contain lots of sugar and harmful chemicals that interfere with your liver functions. I have a small list of processed foods in step 4 of *Automatic Natural Weight Loss System*. Your food choices should be 80% alkaline and 20% acid. Eliminating the acid environment in your body by eating whole foods creates an automatic fat burning machine. This puts less stress on your liver so it can be instrumental in helping to achieve automatic fat burning status.

The two main functions of the liver are to breakdown fats and filter harmful substances (detox) from the blood. If you eliminate or reduce the processed foods from your food choices, your liver can focus on automatic fat burning. There are hundreds of whole food choices you can prepare such as: Fish, eggs, fruits, vegetables, olive oil, rice, potatoes, and more. The point is that these whole foods can be eaten and put less stress on the liver to lose weight. It may be more time consuming in the beginning, but you will learn to organize your time to include better health. Of course, there are pros and cons with each food choice but the main point is to not overwork the liver.

Step 5

Stop counting those calories! Calories do not matter as much as the quality of foods you eat. Your body will tell you when to eat and how much. Always eat until almost full between reasonable hours. Eating after reasonable hours should consist of water type foods such as cucumbers, tomatoes, grapes, lettuce, salads, pineapple, and similar type foods. In fact, when you start eating whole foods again, you will find that you are not eating enough food for calories your body needs. Processed foods are usually high in calories so it makes you full faster on smaller portions.

Imagine if you are eating processed foods what it is really doing to your body. Your body is getting high calorie junk that it cannot assimilate or use so your body is really suffering from a lack of nutrition. This puts your body in a mode of holding on to fat for its survival and it literally robs other parts of the body for nutrients it should be getting from your food choices. This causes a deficiency in nutrients and maintenance of the bones, teeth, skin, organs, and systems of the body. It is a domino effect all from not giving your body whole foods and nutrition. You have an even tougher task of dealing with chemically altered, insecticide, and genetically processed foods. So when you are choosing your foods, choose the highest quality you can afford or grow your own food if possible.

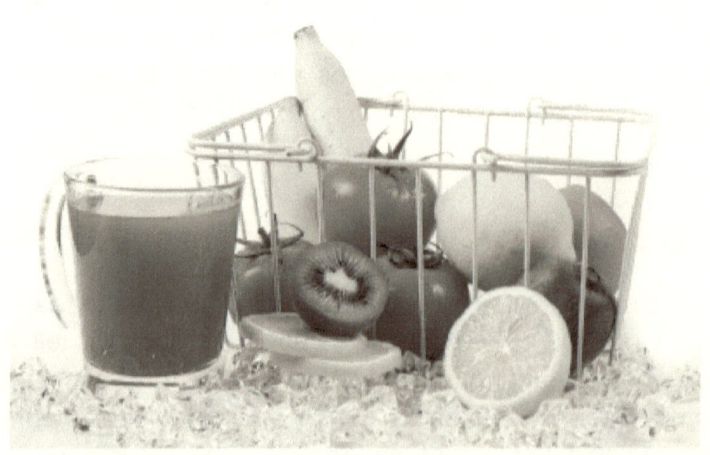

Chapter 6

International Weight Loss Secrets

This section will help give you some tips from around the world that will set your weight loss goals apart from all the other diet programs out there. It gives you an international edge and makes all others look incomplete. This will give you a global view of how weight is controlled, and the global experience of weight loss success. This section can be an addition to step eight of the *Automatic Natural Weight Loss System*. This section focuses on the food consumption and physical aspect of weight loss. This is good because this helps you to adapt to any situation nutritionally that you may come across by giving you international automatic fat burning secrets.

We have chosen certain countries or cultures that have a handle on weight loss and its principles. Eating at the restaurants of these cultures is not the same unless they eliminate or use sparingly the extra sugar, salt, and cheese they use to appeal to you. In order for the international weight loss secrets to be beneficial, it must be traditional without all the additives. These secrets are their traditional views on healthy living that is simple and powerful. Utilize these international weight loss secrets and put your automatic fat burning on turbo. Have fun and open your mind to international weight loss secrets!

1. Mediterranean Secrets- When speaking of the Mediterranean Diet or system, it is important to remember its source of knowledge. Many scholars and historians today are revealing and confirming the Mediterranean Diet is based on principles and habits shared from East Africa namely Ancient Egypt because of how close it is and the documented travels from their most noted historians. **In the Mediterranean, they use olive oil as the main fat.** Olive oil is rich in monounsaturated fats and lowers LDL cholesterol. Drizzling olive oil over dark leafy green vegetables helps you to absorb their Vitamins A, E, and K.

2. Chinese Secrets- Because meat is expensive in rural China, **meat is used as a condiment or as a side dish.** The foundation of their diet is plant foods, rice, and a wide range of vegetables. Meat is seasoning as opposed to the main part of the meal.

3. Japanese Secrets- Japanese start their meals traditionally with soup. Starting your meal with soup is beneficial because it helps with digestion, and decreases overeating with the rest of your meal.

4. Indian Secrets- The people from India maintain their weight by accepting vegetarianism as their diet. Simply speaking, abstaining from meat will eliminate a lot of issues health wise. The cow is actually a sacred animal in India, and it is allowed to roam freely through the streets. Cut the meat, and fat you will defeat.

5. French Secrets- The French eat rich cheese and cured meats washed down with wine and are not obese. How? **Their biggest meal is at lunch, not the beginning or end of the day.** Their portions are small and traditionally they do not snack. When you eat late, you tend to eat fattening things.

6. Mexican Secrets- Traditionally, Mexicans control their blood sugar level, any chance of diabetes, and fat drastically by including certain foods as their staples. **Those staples are squash, beans, and corn.** It is rich in fiber and helps tremendously with the digestive process. This is a pearl for those who have diabetes and want to reverse their condition naturally. Hmmmm.

7. Latin American Secrets- Traditionally Latin Americans take their time, sit down, and eat with family and friends. **Social eating and dining encourages conversation that causes you to usually eat more slowly and eat less.** Your brain needs about twenty minutes to feel satisfied and full. This is accomplished with sitting down and enjoying your meal with family and friends.

8. United States- People from the United States traditionally include nuts as a topping on their meals, or as a healthy snack. It lowers harmful LDL cholesterol and triglycerides (fats) in the blood. Nuts and seeds such as sunflower seeds and pumpkin seeds have tremendous benefits for your weight loss program.

9. African Secrets- Traditionally, Africans made sure whole grains, beans, and fermented foods were the bulk of their food choices. Meat was consumed in small amounts. Millet was a popular whole grain used. These food choices insured a meal in fiber and nutrients. **This kept the blood sugar rate normal and insured a high metabolism for automatic fat burning.**

What have we learned from international food choices around the world? They all have healthy, proven, and factual habits to help maintain and lose weight. If we summarize this into a powerful secret system, it would be:

- **Use Olive oil as your main fat**
- **Start your meals with soup**
- **Limit your meat or eliminate it altogether and become a vegetarian**
- **Make lunch your biggest meal**
- **Include nuts as a topping for your meals or as a healthy snack**
- **Make squash, beans, corn**
- **Fermented foods**
- **A wide range of vegetables**
- **Whole grains as the bulk of your meals.**

If you are part of any of these cultures, it would best serve you and your weight loss goals to adhere to your cultural principles. Your physical body will respond better because it is already in your DNA. I hope the International Weight Loss Secrets will help you even further and broaden your perspective. We can all learn from what has worked globally and what is working globally.

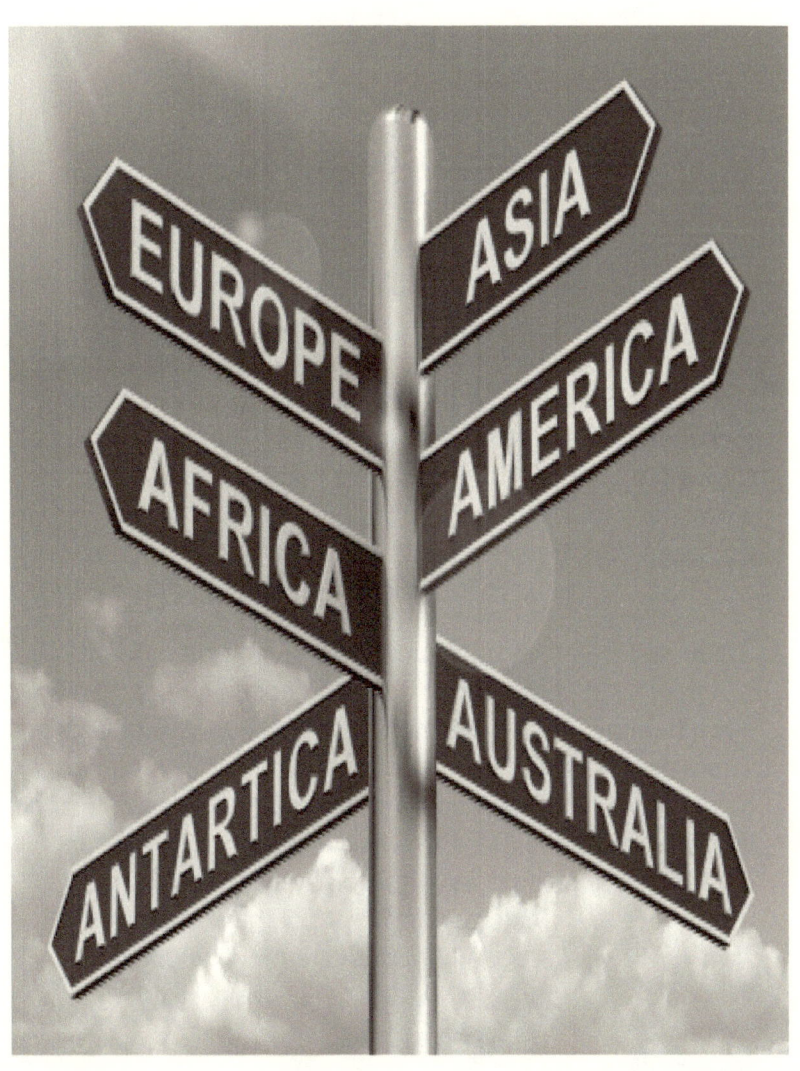

Chapter 7

Food Combining

Many people teach "eat less and exercise more to lose weight." Diet plans tell you to cut back on certain foods and include a certain amount of exercise as part of your program. Food combinations are almost never discussed. How you combine your food choices is very important for digestion and the assimilation process. This is imperative for weight control and weight loss because your body stores less fat cells. An improper food combination confuses your body and puts it on hold until it is figured out. This can result in fat cells being formed.

Steak and potatoes or a hamburger is normal to many, but it is poor food combination. Food combining helps you to eat a healthy and simple meal that gives you more energy. There are many details to food combining which can be a book within itself. I will give you simple principles to include with your food choices so you can have a more efficient digestion that is imperative to weight loss. This helps you with the proper foods part in Step 3 of the *Automatic Natural Weight Loss System* section of this book.

1. Eat fruits alone.

2. Eat proteins with non-starchy foods (i.e. broccoli, cabbage, green beans, lettuces, bok choy, etc.) or ocean vegetables (i.e. kelp, wakame, sea moss, bladder wrack, Irish moss, etc.).

3. Eat grains (i.e. amaranth, spelt, kamut, millet, quinoa, etc) and starchy vegetables (i.e. squash, peas, corn,

artichokes, potatoes, etc) with non-starchy vegetables or ocean vegetables.

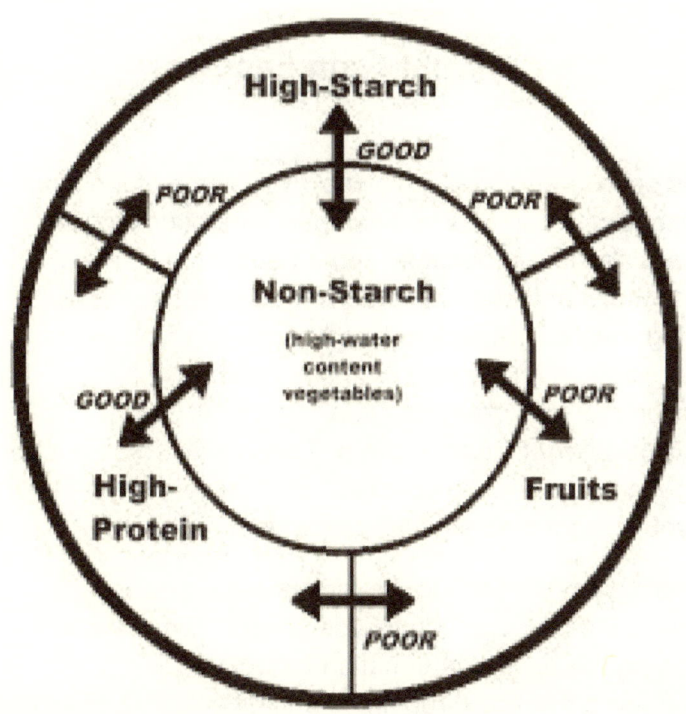

Chapter 8

Weight Gain Factors

This section was created to show you some of the hidden reasons why and how you can gain weight unknowingly. This is necessary because some people may have a perfect diet and exercise program, but still have trouble losing weight. The factors listed below can help assess your situation and work towards reversing the factors. This section provides detail for Step 1 in this *Automatic Natural Weight Loss System.* This is why it is important to get a holistic health consultation or assessment as part of your program so you can see where you stand.

Reversing or eliminating the factors listed below could remove the block for you to lose weight. The value in knowing this type of information far outweighs you purchasing this book 100 times because it is life changing! I will put small notes next to some of the factors that may not be clear. If you think you have one or more of these factors, get with a qualified holistic consultant or doctor that can provide you with holistic remedies and solutions.

Weight Gain Factors:

1. Steroids- cause water weight.

2. Antidepressants- decreases metabolic rate and increases hunger.

3. Diabetes medication

4. Heartburn treatments

5. Birth Control Medication

6. Migraine Relievers

7. Seizure preventatives

8. Going on vacation- normal diet thrown out the window.

9. Working too much- stress can lead to eating.

10. Lack of sleep- body stores fat.

11. Stress

12. Relying on "low-fat" foods

13. Not eating enough fiber- creates a feeling of fullness causing you to eat less.

14. Too much high fructose corn syrup

15. Drinking too many sodas

16. Friends who are overeaters- tend to copy the company you keep.

17. Paying with credit cards at dinner- tend to spend more and eat more.

18. Not eating enough- causes metabolism to lower.

19. Quitting smoking- adjust for the great accomplishment.

20. Small lifestyle changes- change in normal eating and exercise system.

21. New relationship- causes stagnation sometimes.

22. Portion size

23. Spending too much time at the bar

24. Skipping meals

25. Eating too fast- body cannot register it is full

26. Not intensifying your workout routine

27. Menopause- redistribution of weight and greater appetite.

28. Food allergies- cause cravings when you eat it.

29. Aging- causes metabolism to slow down.

30. Feeling guilty- feel guilty about the weight gain and give up.

31. Depression- causes you to eat to satisfy.

32. Getting a cold- certain viruses cause body to hold on to fat cells.

33. Genes

34. Working Out- muscle weight gains first, fat weight lost later.

35. Inflammation

36. Pregnancy

37. Water retention

38. Thyroid problems

39. Cushing's Syndrome

40. Essential Fatty Acid Deficiency

41. Kidney disease

42. Heart trouble

43. Blood Sugar imbalances

44. Ovarian Cysts

45. Tumors

46. Liver dysfunction

47. Fibromyalgia

48. Breast Cancer treatments

49. Adrenal dysfunction

50. Sleep Apnea

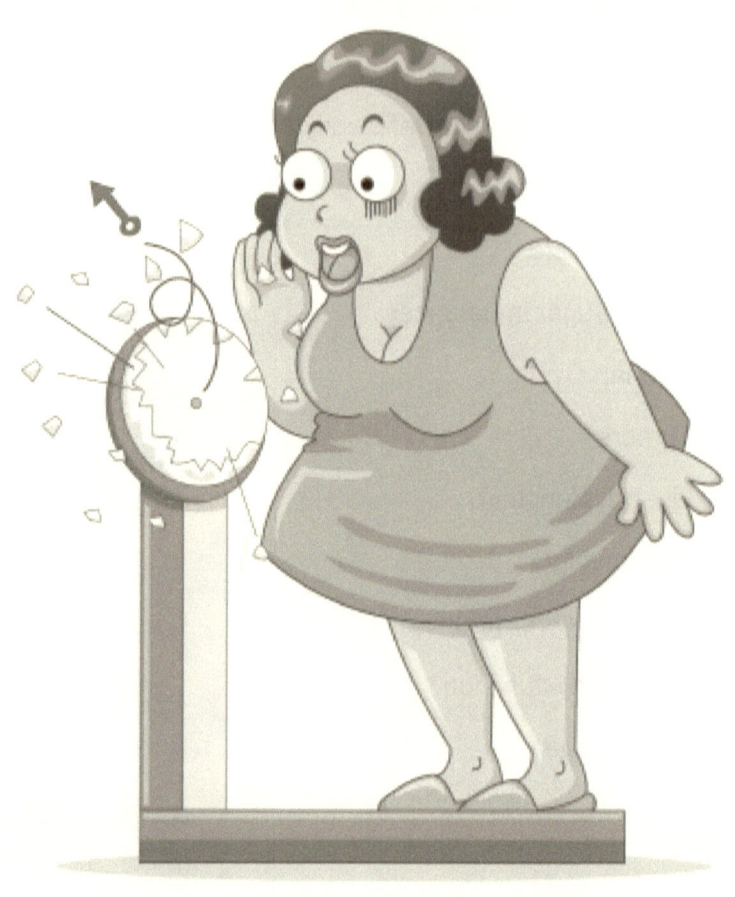

Chapter 9

Holistic Weight Loss and Body Cycles

This is a research study put together last year from various facts gathered through the years that I found very beneficial for excellent health. This research study can be used to enhance your food choices with your weight loss system. You will find this very helpful in your goals. I have had many people apply this research study within their daily life and lose weight the first week. I decided to include this as a bonus to what you have already. Knowing when to eat is just as important as what you eat. Try this and you will experience the results!

Holistic Weight Loss Research Study

This Research study not only results in weight loss, but also a healthier lifestyle. You will notice positive changes overall once you put this plan into practice.

Below are the 3 cycles you should put into practice for optimum health and weight management.

Appropriation noon to 8 p.m. (eating and digestion)

Assimilation 8 p.m. to 4 a.m. (absorption or use)

Elimination 4 a.m. to noon (disposal of body waste and food debris)

When you are awake, you eat (assimilate), and when you are sleeping the body has little other work to do, so it assimilates what it has taken in during the day. The "morning breath" that you have when you get up in the morning is due to the body's elimination cycle.

Before and after designated times, you should only eat water foods, such as fresh fruit, fresh vegetables, salads or any foods that are juicy when bitten into. Water needs no digestion; therefore water foods need very little digesting, and are easy on the system. You may also drink juiced fruits and vegetables, smoothies, and herbal teas with supplements. Solid foods after the times mentioned above need a lot of digesting, thus the digestive system must work harder. Fasting on liquids helps give the body a rest, helps stimulate, and helps cleanse. You can do the same with a fruit fast, vegetable fast, tea fast, etc. This means you would not eat anything except the item you choose to eat (fruit, vegetable, tea, etc). This is powerful and effective because you are still feeding the body necessary nutrients, but you are training the body to accept the proper portions while maintaining or bringing yourself to your natural body weight.

Something as simple as water consumption is very important in weight loss. Drink at least 8 oz. of water 8 times during the day. This helps with digestion and helps eliminate wastes properly. Add Yerba Mate to your diet and see the hunger cravings diminish!

Eat foods that are good to strengthen the liver, kidneys, and pancreas such as alfalfa, apples, apricots, asparagus, bananas, broccoli, cantaloupe, cucumber, cranberry juice, grapes, lemons, limes, melons, squash, yams, etc.

Cut back the dairy (milk, cheese, cream, etc). Animal milk is for animals.

Dieting without daily exercise can cause you to get fatter over time. Find some time each day to include some kind of exercise such as Tai Chi Chuan, walking, exercising, running errands, house chores, etc.

Fast from sunrise to sunset (liquid, fruit, vegetable, yerba mate, etc.) at least one day a week. Make sure you get your daily nutrients by eating a variety of whatever you choose to fast with.

Once a month take a natural laxative (i.e. senna, cascara sagrada, etc.)

Practice all of this to the letter and you will see results within two weeks. Consult doctor or physician before taking on a diet or weight loss program.

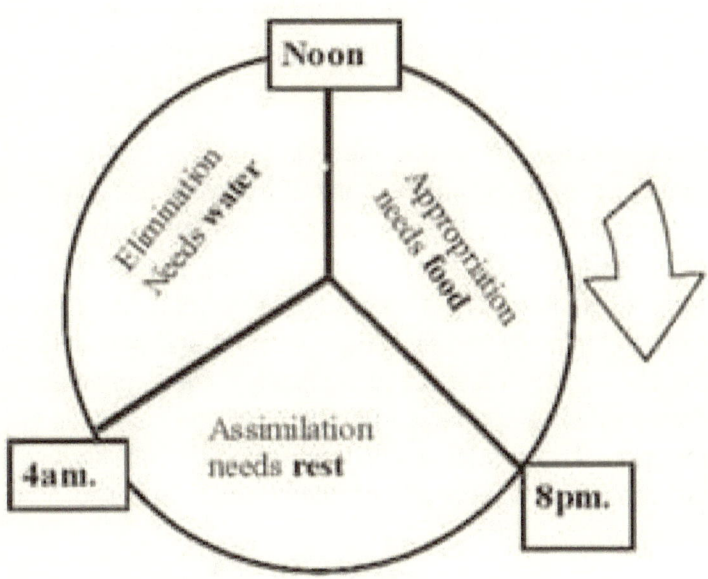

Chapter 10

Holistic Weight Loss System
9 Step Fat Burning System

You are about to begin a system designed to help you lose weight and more importantly burn fat! Go gradually until you get to step nine. What you are doing is putting a system or cycle back in alignment with your body's natural cycles. Fat is not as elusive as most people think. The problem is that most people do not deal with facts as much as they would like to. Two plus two equals four and the earth revolves around the sun. These two facts are not my opinion nor is it a belief. It is a fact! Too many of us simply do not check into the facts or basics of things we hear or read so we are misled.

If we want to lose weight, then why not look at the functions, systems, and organs of the body and learn how it works? If we want to lose weight, why not uncover what causes weight gain naturally in the body and what causes weight loss naturally in the body? Why not uncover what causes the body to gain weight from fat and what causes the body to eliminate fat scientifically? These answers will provide the natural keys to burning fat and losing weight for good! These answers will remove the doubt and eliminate side effects and problems down the road. You will know thyself!

"Know Thyself" is an Ancient Egyptian principle that is the key to our system. Turn inward and learn the keys to your body. Your body is nothing but a microcosm of nature and the universe that is the macrocosm. Nature and the universe is a system designed for balance and so is your body. Most machines and even the automobile are patterned after the human body. You have your organs, systems, and fluids. If you neglect any of the three, it will shut down or not work properly. Now that you have a foundation of what is needed, we will begin to share with you the *Automatic Natural Weight Loss System*. You will be surprised at its simplicity.

Holistic Health Assessment and Consultation

The first action you need to take is to get a holistic health consultation. This is necessary to see in which direction you can go for your fat-burning overhaul. At Living Temple of Life, we have several programs to help you with Holistic Health Consultations. This is important because if you have a certain organ or system that is not functioning properly, this can cause weight gain and pressure on other systems and organs that do work. Next, you will end up taking medication or supplements that can cause weight gain as well. In addition, the holistic assessment & consultation is more important than a regular health assessment & consultation for several reasons.

With a holistic health assessment & consultation, you will get your emotional, spiritual, and mental conditions examined. Consultants may vary in their process or assessment. You should get a blood pressure analysis with your consultation. You will not get a blood pressure test, but an analysis. You should also get a Ph saliva and urine test to check your internal organs and systems. You should get remedies including diet, herbs, music, metals, aromatherapy, and more. It is important because this may be the reason why you take certain actions or non-action each day for your weight loss.

After receiving a good Holistic Health Assessment & Consultation, you will know your strong and weak parts of your whole body. Now you can work specifically on organs and systems that are weak by strengthening them with this program. This will remove the toxins and fat cells and replace it with healthy and vibrant cells. If at all costs you cannot afford to get a holistic health consultation then you can keep in mind past ailments you have had and go with that until you are able to get one. This step is important because it helps in better assessing your overall health situation. It presents the facts so you know exactly what to work with. You are now ready for step 2 of the *Automatic Natural Weight Loss System.*

Colon Cleanse and Detox

The next step is to rid the colon and the rest of your body of any excess waste and toxins. Your holistic health consultation was necessary first so you could see which organs and systems are weak and which ones are not. This will let you know which form of colon cleanse and detox you can take. This is necessary because you do not want to lose weight and fat, and then have waste and toxins remaining in your body. This will ensure that when you lose the fat, your body will rejuvenate itself will real nutrients and not wastes from toxins in your body. Moreover, right now nutrients absorbed into your body feeds the toxic cells in your body keeping them alive. We want to eliminate and starve those cells! I will list below in order of what you can take. For example, if you cannot take Senna or Cascara Sagrada then take the Epsom salt. If you cannot take that, then take Aloe Vera and so forth.

You can cleanse your colon properly by using pure Senna herb (Cassia Senna). The leaves and pods of the Senna plant contain compounds called anthraquinones, which are powerful laxatives. Bowel movements usually occur 6 to 12 hours after taking Senna. Senna should not be used for more than seven consecutive days unless under a doctor's supervision. It should not be used to get a daily bowel movement. Senna or other anthraquinone-containing herbs should not be used by people with diverticular disease, ulcerative colitis, Crohn's disease, severe hemorrhoids, blood vessel disease, congestive heart failure, heart disease, severe anemia, abdominal hernia, gastrointestinal cancer, recent colon surgery, or liver and kidney disease. It should also be avoided if you are pregnant or nursing. Children should not use Senna.

Cascara Sagrada (rhamnus purshiana) is also good. Cascara Sagrada contains compounds called anthraquinones, which are responsible for cascara's powerful laxative effects. Anthraquinones trigger contractions in the colon, called peristalsis, which causes the urge to have a bowel movement. Today, it is one of the most common herbal laxatives. Cascara Sagrada should not be used for longer than 7 days in a row. Pregnant or nursing women should not use Cascara Sagrada. Children should not use Cascara Sagrada. Cascara or other anthraquinone-containing herbs should not be used by people diverticular disease, ulcerative colitis, Crohn's disease, severe hemorrhoids, blood vessel disease, congestive heart failure, heart disease, severe anemia, abdominal hernia, gastrointestinal cancer, recent colon surgery, or liver and kidney disease. It should not be used if appendicitis is suspected. Cascara may interact with drugs called cardiac glycosides, such as digitalis.

If you cannot take Senna or Cascara Sagrada, you can cleanse the colon using Epsom salt. Epsom salt works close as a laxative by a process of hyper osmosis. This means that when Epsom salts are ingested, then they pass through the bowels and attract water molecules from the different parts of the body. This causes the bowels to loosen or soften and facilitate easier excretion. People suffering from constipation, struggle with passage of stool as the waste processed in the bowels is hard. Epsom salt increases the amount of water in the bowels, thereby bringing temporary relief to the person. Epsom salts can be mixed with water and consumed orally, or can be added in a rectal enema. Epsom salt laxative recipe is very simple. All one needs is Epsom salt and some water.

In 8 ounces (1 cup) of drinking water, add approximately 1-2 tsp of Epsom salt. This is just a rough approximation. Check the packet or box of Epsom salt for specific instructions. The amount of Epsom salt added will also vary according to one's age. If you cannot stand the taste of the mixture, simply squeeze a lemon into the Epsom salt solution and drink it. Since the Epsom salt works within the next half an hour, make sure you stay somewhere around the washroom itself. If you do not find relief, repeat the process after an interval of 4 hours. However, do not take more than two doses of Epsom salt solution a day.

Aloe Vera (Aloe Africana) can also be used as a cleanser of the colon. In fact, the FDA has approved Aloe Vera juice as a laxative. You can follow the instructions on the bottle for daily usage. So get some Aloe Vera juice and clean your colon!

Psyllium Whole Husks are also excellent for continually cleansing the colon. A natural plant fiber laxative has special properties. You can take this as long as you prefer and it is even safe for children. You can follow the instructions on the bottle for the amount to use. Drink plenty of water when taking Psyllium whole husks in any form.

Lastly, prune juice is also great as a natural laxative and colon cleanser. These are the keys to achieving the second step in the *Automatic Natural Weight Loss System*. You can actually achieve this in the first three days. This means whichever natural laxative you use to cleanse your colon, you can cleanse for a period of one to three days. You can also switch it up how you like. For example, you can take Senna the first day, Epsom salt the next, and prune juice the last day. You can cleanse for only one day or all three days. To maintain a healthy colon, increase your intake of fiber foods and plenty of water. It is that simple!

Detoxing is such a broad topic with so many opinions, we would like to simplify it for you and just deal with the facts. Detoxing your body simply means to remove the toxins from your blood, organs, tissues, and systems. When toxins accumulate over time, cells mutate and grow until it becomes degenerative such as cancer. You can detox as much as two to three times a year and then stay on a steady program of eating the right foods, drinking cleansing liquids, and maintaining a healthy liver. After all, eliminating toxins is one of the main functions of the liver. Would it be common sense to make sure your liver is always functioning properly so it can do its job? You can find a good detox package that takes care of all of these things. Most detox packages are consumed over a period of one week on up to a month. In essence, you may still be detoxing while you are on the Automatic **Natural Weight Loss System**. This is good because you will be eliminating the cycle of fat and toxins while you lose the weight. After one to three days of cleansing the colon and starting your detox program, your body will be ready to go to step three of the **Automatic Natural Weight Loss System**.

Proper Exercise, Proper Breathing, Proper Relaxation, Positive Thinking, and Proper Foods

This step is necessary to put your body within a natural system of health and maintenance. This alone will help you burn fat cells and improve your overall health. This step will be more difficult to include within your life but the key is to include a little at a time. You have to start with one-step at a time. That is the natural cycle of things and growth. You cannot plant seeds and expect them to naturally grow overnight. Likewise, you have to take your time with this step. Even if you include each part of this step for five minutes then it is a start. You can work your way up to spending more time with each step over time. The key is to stick with it because anything you do for 30 consecutive days becomes a habit whether it is good or bad.

Proper Exercise is paramount in this system. The most natural and best exercise you can do is to walk. Walking as an exercise for at least 30 minutes a day will do wonders for your body. It will help burn those fat cells and it increases your metabolism. If you walk properly and naturally briskly, you will tone your whole body. You can get it in other ways too if you cannot do it continuously for 30 minutes a day. If you go to the store, park far at the end of the parking lot. Take the stairs instead of the elevator. Something is better than nothing, and it starts the 30-day habit. Soon your body will not feel right unless you walk and exercise. If you want to remove fat from certain areas of your body, do exercises specific for those areas. This is not the arena for discussing what is correct or not. There is ample information out there to address it, but you want to make sure you do exercise regularly (3-5 days a week). Unlike a regular schedule of exercise limited to 3-5 days a week, you can exercise walk everyday!

Proper Breathing is very important because it helps give oxygen to your organs and systems. It also helps remove toxins from the body. Breathing properly gives you natural vitality necessary to give you the energy to be more active that can help increase your metabolism. You should do some form of deep breathing everyday to charge your whole system. There is a wealth of information on deep breathing and it is like recharging your battery. You will be surprised at how beneficial just 5 minutes of deep breathing a day is for your overall health. From now on, practice deep breathing at least 5 minutes a day.

Proper Relaxation is the natural opposite of work and activity. You must have true rest and relaxation to counteract stress. Every piece of good machinery has a rest period. Relaxation is not going on a vacation. Usually, all kinds of depressants and stimulants are pumped into your body in many different ways. Learn to settle down or even meditate. The key is to relax your nerves every day. That is why massage parlors are so successful these days. People refuse to get proper rest and relaxation that can burn you out which also helps the energy drink industry. It all works hand in hand. You want to step outside of that trap and just relax each day, and get some "me" time. Proper relaxation can be done by meditating, sitting in a quiet place for a time that is good for you, resting/sleeping, and anything thing else that brings you away from stimulants and movement of the body.

Positive Thinking will give you the drive to continue with this program. It is the key to getting you through each day. Thought is energy and you can send or receive these waves. That is why you can walk into a room after an argument and know an argument took place. The opposite is walking into a room after a party and know that one took place. You can create your fortune just by your thoughts, just as some people think themselves into a cold! That is also why motivational speakers are needed, as well as rallies for sports teams. It is all about your positive thinking. Practice it every chance you get. Do not identify with negative thoughts, gossip, slander, jealousy, envy, and hatred. You will get the full benefit of positive thinking.

Proper Foods are necessary for any weight loss program because you will need the foods that do not encourage or put you in a position to create fat cells. You want to stay away from processed foods, fast foods, sugar foods, and salty foods as often as possible. Just those alone cause most of the problem in many ways for creating and feeding fat cells. Simply work your nutrition around that and you will see an immediate difference in your health and fat cells will start to suffocate and die. pH balance is a real key in your food choices and program. Proper pH puts the body in a position to assimilate or utilize more of the nutrients from your food choices. Eating for pH balance is the key to metabolizing the nutrients from the foods you eat. Your food choices should be 80% alkaline and 20% acid. This creates an environment for automatic fat burning. Re-read this part because you might miss how simple it is.

Incorporate this system in your daily regimen and you will start to take off in your 9 Step fat burning system. Do not overwhelm yourself and lose track. Remember if you just do a little of each every day, it will increase over time like a snowball effect. This is another of the steps that will continue throughout your program of losing the fat cells. You have now had the opportunity to implement 3 of the 9 steps of the *Automatic Natural Weight Loss System.*

Eliminate or Replace Bad Food

What is bad food? Research what happened to a small island paradise called Naru and you will see what bad food does to a whole population. Bad food is food that has very little or no nutritional value for your body. Bad food would include white flour, white sugar, white bread, white salt, processed food, fast food, sugary foods, salty foods, frozen foods and bad fruits and vegetables. The list also includes artificial sweeteners, microwavable foods, diet health bars & products, and processed soy products. Of course, I am stepping on many feet by mentioning these bad foods... especially economic feet. This food only settles in the body and turns into fat cells or causes you to overeat that can do the same thing.

Once you replace your nutrition with healthy and fresh foods, you will see a difference in your body and it will be less stress on your liver. Proper nutrition feeds healthy cells and replenishes your energy when needed. This step is simple and can be practiced at any time and for the duration of the program. Some people just practice this step alone and lose fat cells because this step is so simple yet powerful. It will happen automatically! Almost everywhere you go, unhealthy food choices are everywhere so you must bring healthy food choices with you to compensate. This does not mean you cannot ever eat at a fast food restaurant or eat something processed. It just means you need to eat well at least 90% of the time and leave room for splurge within reason. Within reason, means do not go out and eat a baby pig or five Big Macs at once.

Read those labels and change your food choices and you will see the crap literally leave your system! It may cost a little more for each item, but your health is worth it right? You may have to give most of your food in your refrigerator, freezer, and pantry away. You may have to start from scratch but it will be the biggest move you have ever made in your automatic fat burning goals. Once you incorporate this step, you are well on your way to lose the fat cells more rapidly because now they will starve to death. Step 5 is next and ready to upload into your nine step automatic fat burning system.

Emotional Weight Loss

How can you talk about losing weight or fat when you do not address how people eat emotionally? Your emotions can get heavy or "fat" and needs to shed the weight if it is out of shape. Your emotions are love, hate, grief, compassion, jealousy, concern, envy, worry, depression, happiness, kindness, respect, care, and more. The negative emotions need curtailing or elimination from your life. When you let negative emotions govern your life, it affects your physical body because most people eat emotionally.

Most do not eat for nutrition. Instead, they eat how they feel right now. If you lose your boyfriend or girlfriend, people sometimes resort to eating, drinking, or drug use.

Some people eat things they know they should not all the time, but do not have the discipline to stop. The key is to focus on the opposite and become active. Meaning if any negative emotion arises, do some kind of action such as exercise, do a hobby, help someone, read, watch a good movie, and more. Since emotions are symbolic of stemming from the heart, it is also symbolic of the gas or breath of life.

Your emotions are from the soul, it is the real you. The heart symbolically resembles a flame or fire. Even old girlfriends or boyfriends are "my old flame", and fire gives off gas. So if you need to lose that weight on your soul, try deep breathing or meditating more and you will see your soul and emotions will be less heavy with negativity or extra weight. This step is a work in progress as you consistently work at it constantly until it becomes a good habit. This will help you lose weight physically because it will help you to eat from a nutrition standpoint instead of an emotional standpoint. It will also free your emotions for higher or lighter vibrations to others and it will be felt pleasantly. Lose that fat emotionally!

Spiritual Weight Loss

Is your spiritual body fat? Your spiritual body is your personality and the fluid or water part of you. Your emotions generate from within and equate feelings, but the spirit is mainly what you issue out or give. For example, your personality (spiritual) loves towards (fluid, water) others, while you have an emotion (gas, fire, burning) of love. Do you have excess spiritual weight? Excess spiritual weight means you do not share yourself with others or you do not give back. So in essence, your personality becomes selfish. Selfishness is "spiritual laziness" to many people. The remedy to this is "As you were given, you now must give."

Let your personality flow with others and the excess weight will fall off because you will raise your spiritual metabolism. That means you will be more active in giving of yourself and your spirit will work more. Is it a coincidence certain phrases "spiritual work", "spiritual exercise" or "spiritual warrior" exists? All of this spiritual work will help you to improve your personality and make better choices for burning fat by giving more than receiving.

Since the spirit flows and moves like water, your liquid intake is essential. You should make sure your water intake is regular because it will help remove the toxins and wastes from the body, as well as help with the function of all your organs and systems of the body. Alkaline or Kangen Water, natural spring water (fresh spring), or well water is better than our water choices on the market. Lose the spiritual weight and let your spiritual body become more attractive. Now you are losing weight and fat beyond a physical level. This is the real meaning of holistic health and weight loss. You see weight or fat can still manifest beyond the physical, and it works hand in hand with the physical body. Now it is time to address the mental weight loss.

Mental Weight Loss

Thought is very powerful and has weight, shape, and size. Mental deals with the mind and thoughts. Every step starts with a thought. Before you made that decision to eat or exercise, you thought about it first. So actually mental fat burning and weight loss is just as important as physical weight loss! You are fat mentally when you have too much on your mind, think improperly, and experience memory loss. Mental fatness mainly deals with being stagnant or inactive mentally. An example of what I am expressing is You have love emotionally, yet spiritually share love with others you meet with, and mentally love occupies your thoughts at times.

The mind is something that is not tangible like the brain, but it is "tapped" into for thoughts, ideas, and inspiration. The exchange between the brain and mind happens by electricity and magnetism. There are 12 cranial nerves and 33 spinal nerves that work with a sympathetic and parasympathetic system. That is why whenever they show an idea or thought; they always show a light bulb that is symbolic of energy or electricity. Your mind and thoughts must be electric! If your thoughts are not fresh and electric, then you are fat mentally and need to lose that weight that is bogging you down.

The key to losing the mental fat is to feed it properly and exercise it often and regularly. How can one accomplish this? You can include foods such as fish, flax seed, or omega 3's. These foods are categorized as brain food. You can also take certain herbs to help such as Gingko Biloba, Hawthorn, Schisandra, Gotu Kola, and Rosemary. Another way to burn the mental fat is to exercise the mind by doing things that cause you to think more than usual such as chess, puzzles, games, and mind benders.

Anything that causes you to think, focus, and remember will strengthen your mental body and help you burn the unwanted stagnant mental energy that settled which is called fat. This will automatically help put your mind and thoughts in order. You have now gotten the keys to physical, emotional, spiritual, and mental fat burning at this point. Applying as many of these steps as possible will bring tremendous results as we embark upon step 8 of our automatic fat burning system.

Culture and Family

Embracing your culture and family is a hidden key to automatic fat burning these days. If you get to the root of most cultures today, you will encounter a system or way of life that is active and uplifting. This gets you involved in something greater than yourself and encourages selflessness instead of selfishness. Your family is your support group because they, along with your friends, will give you the feedback necessary to continue with your automatic fat burning goals. Learn to interact with family and friends about your holistic body and the changes they notice. They can tell you things you may not see or notice about yourself. Sometimes it takes someone on the outside to tell you what is going on in the inside.

Embracing more of your culture helps you to learn more about you and apply the necessary points in your life. Embracing your culture and family gives you the opportunity to lose the extra-unwanted weight because you will be preoccupied with the extra movement. With this extra movement, fat does not get a chance to settle. This step is simple as far as a measuring rod for you. It allows you to see improvements needed, and the direction on which *Automatic Natural Weight Loss System* is working for you. Embrace this step and you will see your metabolism increase just from the extra activity, and it will be your very own support group. Every good cause needs a strong support team to continue forward.

Renew and Share

This is the final step in the *Automatic Natural Weight Loss System*! You have a wealth of no nonsense and practical guidelines for automatic fat loss. You should feel a lot better right now and have more energy. Some of you may see that some of your other ailments have subsided too. This system on average takes at least 30 days to complete, but it may take some people longer to complete and others shorter. The key is to instill the system in your life. Some steps may be harder than other steps, but you can definitely accomplish it. The key is to constantly renew or review the steps until it becomes a habit in your life. These positive habits will cause fat to run when it comes near you. You will also know how to solve any fat problem quickly and practically upon finishing reading this book.

Each week or each month do yourself a favor and renew or review this system to see what you are still doing correctly and what you need to work on. If you keep renewing this system, you will have formed good habits to lose fat automatically in nine simple steps. You are obligated to share this system with others so they can also do the same thing you did. This means having them get their own *Automatic Natural Weight Loss System* book so they can lose the unwanted fat safely and naturally too. You were given, so now you must give. Keep the balance. This will put you in the status of completion.

The reason step 9 is "renew and share" points to what is natural in our numbers. Nine is a symbol of birth because after nine the numbers start over again. This is a natural cycle of birth, growth, reproduction, and renewal. Therefore, this system of automatic fat burning is complete once you continue and repeat the process until it becomes first nature again. You will now get a bonus of supporting material that is just as important as the *Automatic Natural Weight Loss System* you just completed. This supporting chart compliments the *Automatic Natural Weight Loss System* for even faster and naturally holistic results. The key is "know thyself" and put your holistic body back into its natural cycle. There is no need for drugs, chemicals, medicine, operations, or surgery.

ALKALIZING FOODS			ACIDIFYING FOODS		
VEGETABLES	**FRUITS**	**OTHER**	**FATS & OILS**	**NUTS & BUTTERS**	**DRUGS & CHEMICALS**
Garlic	Apple	Apple Cider Vinegar	Avocado Oil	Cashews	Chemicals
Asparagus	Apricot	Bee Pollen	Canola Oil	Brazil Nuts	Drugs, Medicinal
Fermented Veggies	Avocado	Lecithin Granules	Corn Oil	Peanuts	Drugs, Psychedelic
Watercress	Banana (high glycemic)	Probiotic Cultures	Hemp Seed Oil	Peanut Butter	Pesticides
Beets	Cantaloupe	Green Juices	Flax Oil	Pecans	Herbicides
Broccoli	Cherries	Veggies Juices	Lard	Tahini	
Brussel sprouts	Currants	Fresh Fruit Juice	Olive Oil	Walnuts	**ALCOHOL**
Cabbage	Dates/Figs	Organic Milk	Safflower Oil		Beer
Carrot	Grapes	(unpasteurized)	Sesame Oil	**ANIMAL PROTEIN**	Spirits
Cauliflower	Grapefruit	Mineral Water	Sunflower Oil	Beef	Hard Liquor
Celery	Lime	Alkaline Antioxidant Water		Carp	Wine
Chard	Honeydew Melon	Green Tea	**FRUITS**	Clams	
Chlorella	Nectarine	Herbal Tea	Cranberries	Fish	**BEANS & LEGUMES**
Collard Greens	Orange	Dandelion Tea		Lamb	Black Beans
Cucumber	Lemon	Ginseng Tea	**GRAINS**	Lobster	Chick Peas
Eggplant	Peach	Banchi Tea	Rice Cakes	Mussels	Green Peas
Kale	Pear	Kombucha	Wheat Cakes	Oyster	Kidney Beans
Kohlrabi	Pineapple		Amaranth	Pork	Lentils
Lettuce	All Berries	**SWEETENERS**	Barley	Rabbit	Lima Beans
Mushrooms	Tangerine	Stevia	Buckwheat	Salmon	Pinto Beans
Mustard Greens	Tomato		Corn	Shrimp	Red Beans
Dulce	Tropical Fruits	**SPICES/SEASONINGS**	Oats (rolled)	Scallops	Soy Beans
Dandelions	Watermelon	Cinnamon	Quinoi	Tuna	Soy Milk
Edible Flowers		Curry	Rice (all)	Turkey	White Beans
Onions	**PROTEIN**	Ginger	Rye	Venison	Rice Milk
Parsnips (high glycemic)	Eggs	Mustard	Spelt		Almond Milk
Peas	Whey Protein Powder	Chili Pepper	Kamut	**PASTA (WHITE)**	
Peppers	Cottage Cheese	Sea Salt	Wheat	Noodles	
Pumpkin	Chicken Breast	Miso	Hemp Seed Flour	Macaroni	
Rutabaga	Yogurt	Tamari		Spaghetti	
Sea Veggies	Almonds	All Herbs	**DAIRY**		
Spirulina	Chestnuts		Cheese, Cow	**OTHER**	
Sprouts	Tofu (fermented)	**ORIENTAL VEGETABLES**	Cheese, Goat	Distilled Vinegar	
Squashes	Flax Seeds	Maitake	Cheese, Processed	Wheat Germ	
Alfalfa	Pumpkin Seeds	Daikon	Cheese, Sheep	Potatoes	
Barley Grass	Tempeh (fermented)	Dandelion Root	Milk		
Wheat Grass	Squash Seeds	Shitake	Butter		
Wild Greens	Sunflower Seeds	Kombu			
Nightshade Veggies	Millet	Reishi			
	Sprouted Seeds	Nori			
	Nuts	Umeboshi			
		Wakame			
		Sea Veggies			

Charts

The following charts are for you to make and keep a record of your progress. It is a known fact that those who keep track of their progress often succeed more times than not. It helps you to make what you are learning as a habit in your holistic health life. Below I have included brief explanations of how to use your charts. Take advantage of these charts because it helps you solidify everything you have just learned. Please make copies and use as often as needed. Show yourself you are serious!

Foods With No Extra Sugar or Salt

Create a chart that lists the foods or brands that do not have excess sugar/salt in them. Leave a space for you to list how many milligrams/grams of sugar/salt is in the item. This chart is helpful because it helps you to keep track of the food products that do not contain extra salt or sugar. Salt and sugar in excess are the main culprits in weight gain. So when you find a certain item that you like to eat, just find the brand that is the safest for you to eat and log it on your chart. This eliminates you having to read the label of all the foods each time you go shopping. In addition, your body is accustomed to eating certain foods, and it adapts to the healthier choice. It makes your grocery shopping a lot easier and it creates a good habit along the way.

Weekly Meal Plan

Create a weekly chart that allows you to log meals for breakfast, lunch, and dinner. List the beginning and ending weight, blood pressure, pulse, etc. if possible. It should look like a regular calendar. You can even use a calendar. This chart is helpful because you can plan your meals either for the day or for the week. You can also keep track of what you have eaten through the day or week. Either way, it helps you to see all that you are eating so you can include or exclude certain foods in your daily meals. It is something about looking at what you have done. It is a great way to stay encouraged by visually seeing your path. Remember, it is best to curtail the appetite by eating water foods before 11 a.m. and after 9 p.m.

Weekly Goals

Create a chart that allows you to fill in details for the categories of: emotional, mental, spiritual, physical, and financial. This chart is good because it helps you to organize your life by organizing your holistic health. Imagine the possibilities of balanced health. Plan each day to bring your holistic body back in balance. Do something for your emotional body, spiritual body, mental body, and physical body each day. If you do not know what I mean then go back over the sections in this book that explains it.

Do not worry; I did not leave out the financial goals. Have you ever heard the phrase "your health is your wealth"? That phrase is literal and very true. Take care of your health (holistic body) and your wealth is automatic. With a strong emotional body, imagine the vibration and magnetism you will have. With a strong mental body, imagine the ideas that will come to you. With a strong spiritual body, imagine the networking and service you will do. With a strong physical body, the longevity and energy needed to carry out all your needs from your whole body. Anything you put out such as time, energy, or finances for your development and growth, comes back to you in more abundance. It is a universal law.

Postword

I have just presented the hottest, newest, and most complete system for you to lose weight. The great thing about it is you do not have to waste a lot of money on expensive products or classes. In addition, you achieved this weight loss naturally and holistically. The most important way to address your health concerns is to not cover it up and treat the symptoms. You must confront and deal with it head on by addressing its cause. This will start rejuvenating the faulty condition, organ, or system.

In this case, we are dealing with obesity or being overweight. Digestive organs not functioning properly and/or overeating usually cause this. If the liver and pancreas are weak, excess fat accumulates around the abdominals and excess protein becomes fat. Overeating and a diet of junk foods can contribute to this effect. Excess weight (fat) is actually extra cells maintained by the body. These fat cells not only steal energy that is for immunity, but these fat cells are also homes for toxic waste. These cells increase as the organs' functions decrease. These cells also stop the body's abilities to cleanse and maintain health.

The mechanism controlling your appetite can be imbalanced by emotional stress, physical issues with your organs, spiritual issues, or mental problems. This is the reason why this book was necessary in order to address this holistically. Fat cells can choke healthy cells and accumulate waste, toxins, and fat. This decreases the healthy cell life and alters the path of nutrients. This path would go to healthy cells, but instead it goes to fat cells. In essence, obesity is the result of nutrient starvation and disease. It is important to put your body in a position to assimilate proper nutrients.

I am interested in your weight loss testimonials so email me your success! I will post some of your testimonials in our next revised edition. Also, call or email if you would like a seminar or lecture for your church, synagogue, mosque, organization, group, or event. After reading this book, I am sure you can agree that everyone needs to have this information. Thank you for supporting this book and good health!

About the Author

Franklin Gillette

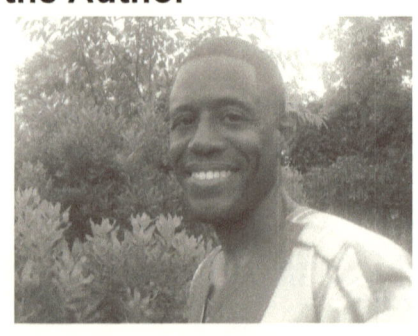

Franklin Gillette is a Nutrition Consultant, Herbalist, Visionary, Author, Humanitarian, Entrepreneur, and Motivational Speaker. Franklin specializes in helping people restore good health naturally according to the laws of health and life. Franklin also values the opportunity to bring out the best in people. He has been on this spiritual path since 1989 progressing, experiencing and sharing the principles of Love, Justice, Balance, Compatibility, Truth, Peace, Freedom, Joy, and Success.

Many people experience him as a very knowledgeable and captivating speaker. When you hear him speak, you will feel motivated to accomplish your goals and learn some of the things you always wanted to know concerning health, love, and abundance. You are sure to add increase to your life from the many books that Franklin has written on numerous topics. He also provides consultation and coaching on all levels for truth and balance.

allowoneness@gmail.com

One Last Thing

I appreciate you reading this wonderful book of mine. The highest thanks you can give me is leaving a review on the site or venue you bought this from (Lulu, iBookstore, Nook, etc.), and referring my book(s) to family and friends.
Thank you!

Franklin Gillette
allowoneness@gmail.com

Why is this book important? Compatibility The Code of Harmony For Love & Unity is important because it is the most comprehensive book ever written on relationships. It looks at relationships from more angles than any book today. This book is the education and training that everyone should get worldwide because it gives you the ability to solve problems. Every problem in the world is lack of compatibility and people not having the proper relationship with themselves. This in turn makes it nearly impossible to have a proper relationship with others. This book gives you the knowledge and ability to help yourself..., which allows you to help others. Learning how to unlock the code of compatibility will give you the keys to open the doors to greater Love, Health, & Abundance!

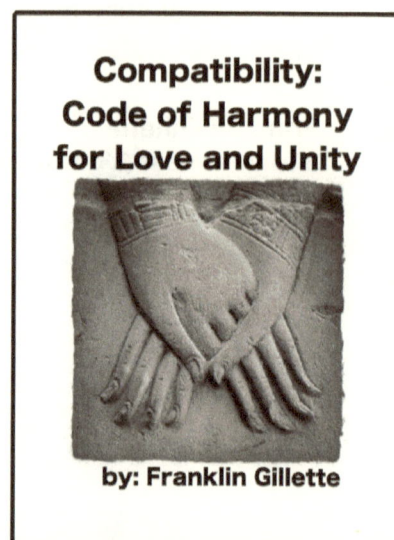

**Compatibility:
Code of Harmony
for Love and Unity**

by: Franklin Gillette

eBook $6.99

soft cover $14.99

This book is for the individual, single mother, student, disabled, elderly, family, group, and community. If you want to ensure a safe environment for yourself or family, then this book has the potential of possibly saving your life! It is not meant to live and walk around in a fearful state of mind. However, it is very wise to do all you practically can to build a strong defense and fortress for protection. Even if you are confident in your security measures, you can this book to someone you love who may not be as prepared. You cannot be everywhere at all times, so it helps to have everyone on the same page to ensure a safe environment mentally and physically. Unless you live in a bubble, this book is a necessary book that you should have and implement into your daily lives. Each chapter focuses on an action that could ease your mind of losing someone or something dear to you.

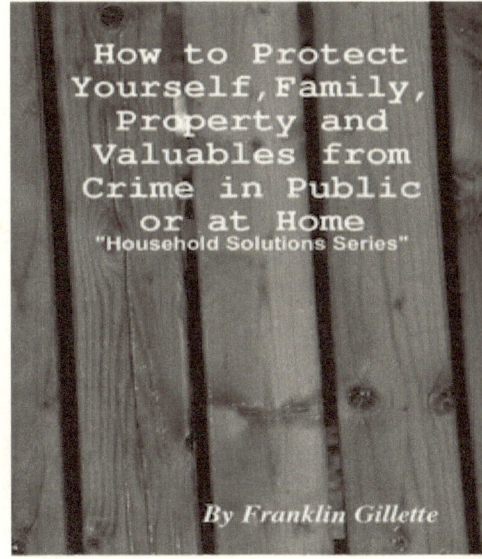

How to Protect Yourself, Family, Property and Valuables from Crime in Public or at Home
"Household Solutions Series"

By Franklin Gillette

eBook $1.99
soft cover coming soon!

Order this book and other titles:
http://www.lulu.com/spotlight/fenex9atyahoodotcom

www.ingramcontent.com/pod-product-compliance
Lightning Source LLC
Chambersburg PA
CBHW020350290526
45785CB00005B/2217